Six Months of Grace

Six Months of Grace

✦

No Time To Die

Raymond S Glover, B.S., RN,
Edited by M. Loreas Powell

iUniverse, Inc.
New York Lincoln Shanghai

Six Months of Grace
No Time To Die

iUniverse books may be ordered through booksellers or by contacting:

iUniverse
2021 Pine Lake Road, Suite 100
Lincoln, NE 68512
www.iuniverse.com
1-800-Authors (1-800-288-4677)

ISBN: 0-595-34072-5

Printed in the United States of America

Twas grace that taught my heart to fear and grace my fear relieved.
-Amazing Grace-

God has raised from death our Lord Jesus, who is the Great Shepherd of the
sheep as the result of his blood, by which the eternal covenant is sealed. May the
God of peace provide you with every good thing you need in order to do his will,
and may he, through Jesus Christ, do in us what pleases him. And to Christ be
the glory forever and ever! Amen.
-Hebrews 13:20–21-

Contents

Acknowledgements

(YOU KNOW WHO YOU ARE)

GOD,
BMLGPADPGLAPJRPAPBJTSSCSTHVLJJSHASJBJBKFGTT-
AMECVFBMAGM
DLYRGNGDLMCPCSCMARSHALLWFEFPFAFBRFGCHCHCHJMSMC-
FRECMLM
LRAEERAYDFJLLGTWVPJBFSWSHERCHRW

Synopsis

In 1997, I was given six months to live and as I now write this book in 2004, each successive doctor has given me that SAME six months' prognosis. While I am not mocking the diagnosis (because one day it will come true), the only reason I am still here is because of God's grace and His will for the information that I need to give to you.

This book is about how I manage the disease. It is my experience. It is not definitive for every one and you should always check your doctor before trying anything. It provides recipes and other Sarcoidosis references. It is a great resource to add to your library or to give to someone who has been struggling with the disease. There are more of us than you know. Look for them, read about what they have, see how you can help and be a friend.

1

"Mr. Glover, you have a serious problem. You need to see an Optometrist immediately." The O.D. examined me and said those words that I amid millions of other diagnosed patients have heard and dread…these words would haunt me and fill me with dread and be a bane to me for the rest of my life……" You have Sarcoidosis". The world came to a screeching halt and the water began covering my head just as the fluid from Sarcoidosis fills your lungs and blocks your lymph nodes to the eyes, making everything dim, suffocating you and leaving you gasping for air. I was grasping for air, trying to process this information and the affect that it was to have on my life. As with other individuals, my life has drastically changed. Sometimes late at night I think that hindsight is twenty-twenty. And I just try to imagine some tell-tale sign, or was there something I could of seen that could of given me an insight given me an inkling of the devastation that this disease would play in my life. I think about that time during a job interview, the flash of the camera hurt my eyes. I remember thinking "this was very strange." But after all, I had never had pink-eye to this extent. I had pink-eye two weeks before, in my left eye. I never thought about it, I just figured, eye infection "no big deal"; then it went into my right eye. I thought that was unusual….just got finished with one eye and then it goes into the other. When that was over and I went to a job interview, the flash made my eyes hurt. I thought, "This was interesting. But it didn't lead me to think of anything major. The Pink-Eye disappeared, and life went on for me. I remember shortly after that that my eyes seemed to not take in so much light. People in my church had this phrase when they got older, the "eyes go dim". I thought that this was what I was experiencing, only WAY, WAY before my time. They often referred to in their prayers and old songs from old hymns.

Now this revelation, in the actual naming of this disease, it was a much similar experience to other Sarcoid patients. "What the hell is Sarcoidosis?" So the doc explained it. I'm a nurse and I was absolutely in denial about having this condition, I said "Yeah, right" with all of the sarcasm that I could muster. "You're telling me that I have a devastating disease that no one knows about and it goes throughout my body and in my eyes but it is supposed to be affecting all of my organs?" "Ok!" and then to top it off, he told me that it was a cousin to Lupus.

Lupus!! Now, I knew what Lupus was and as one of my hobbies was research. I had researched Lupus a long time ago and as I recalled, mostly women contracted Lupus!! So if this was true, then how could I contract this disease called "Sarcoidosis" if I was a male? Disbelief flooded my body. I couldn't grasp what was being told to me. But he confirmed it, gave me medicine for my eyes, I used it. Now let me digress.

My eyes got better and I thought that life was GREAT (ergo NORMAL). This was the summer of 1984. The year that my little brother graduated from Central High School in Georgia and two years after my only sister graduated from the same school. I was young, handsome, and athletic and thought that I had everything going for me....and....I did. There was no way that I believed that there was something lurking within me, waiting to steal my youth, my sight, my oxygen and eventually my life. The only other indicator that this was a real disease for me was when I tried to join the military. I was disqualified for having enlarged lymph nodes and this was a new experience because I didn't know what my lymph nodes were for but that was an indicator. I brushed that off as the Army's loss. It was just less headache for me to not join the military anyway. I was read and disciplined and I just knew that by joining, I would impress the ladies, serving my country was somewhere on the list also. But it was not to be with the discovery; I moved on with my life. I would learn much later that interdisciplinary skills that I had would be far more valuable in the fight against Sarcoidosis than in any position the military would provide for me.

2

Official Diagnosis

In 1987, I moved to New York and then I began notice changes within me. Once again, I was having vision problems. Enrolled in college and studying and unbeknownst to me, I was having trouble. Definitely denial! When I finally realized that I needed glasses, it was astonishing to me to know how bad my sight was and how little regard I had for taking care of it. I would sit in the back of classrooms and have trouble reading the writing on the blackboard. Anyone else might have thought that this was a problem but in my vanity, there was no problem until a friend of mine let me use his or her glasses. Immediately, I saw how much I was missing. I was being given clues and was not to pay attention to them yet. I went to another ophthalmologist to get glasses and that's when I was again informed (this can be considered a second opinion, I think) that I had a condition "There is something wrong with your eyes you have Uveitis". I am very fortunate, unlike many other individuals with Sarcoidosis, I have had the benefit of physicians and other health professionals who recognized the disease very early in its stages. I was the one who denied that this particular disease existed. The informed me that this tiger did exist and was hunting and stalking me. Other people have a condition that they know that is devastating and then they have to inform the doctors and then the doctors do not believe them. My situation was exactly the opposite; I felt no type of symptoms. I was not tired. The eye condition was the only red flag for me. I had to accept the fact that I had this disease and it had devastating consequences. The fact became very evident while I was attending Nursing School. One class exercise was to learn how to take pulse and blood pressure. I discovered during this activity, that I had an irregular pulse. I thought nothing of it, when my teacher checks my pulse, to verify the findings, her reaction was unsuppressed alarm. She forced me to get a signed affidavit from the doctor saying that this was not a life threatening condition. This was so irritating but it was alarmingly apparent to me that there was truly something in my body that was causing problems and I needed to face it.

I began to indulge in my researching hobby and found that many people in the health-care field (at this time) were not aware of this condition. Fortunately, I found some knowledgeable health care providers. I received an official diagnosis of Sarcoidosis in 1987 by Lung Biopsy (Outpatient). My recovery was smooth, I just couldn't drink water. Then I saw a Pulmonary Specialist and upon examination of the x-rays, determined that my lungs had been compromised by the Sarcoid. There was scarring in my lungs. There was scar tissue present. During the pulmonary tests, he showed me the normal levels or respiratory function and compared to my levels. It was pretty obvious that my lung capacity was diminished.

3

Medical Regime and the RIGGAMAROLL

I started the medical regime of 60 mg of Prednisone a day. I thought that I knew the ends and outs of Prednisone until I actually started taking the medication. I was exercising until I found that my weight gain was increasing, TREMEDOUSLY! The reason that I was gaining weight came to me, it was the Prednisone…steroid. It was causing my body to retain fluid. This was upsetting because I ballooned past normal so much to the point where I could not fit into my clothing. The weight gain was fast and furious. On top of this people started making jokes that I was eating the kitchen sink. "Fat jokes", society calls them. I did have an increase in appetite. I was voracious but this was also a side affect of this medication. But my food intake did not warrant this amount of weight. I started to experience memory loss. I spoke with the doctor and he reassured me that these side affects would go away eventually but I required monitoring for the first six months. At this time, I was still thinking that I had an acute condition. This was short term…short lived. The medical regime philosophy was to treat the Sarcoidosis for the best prognosis. It will go into remission upon treatment and then we will take it from there. It wasn't until much later that I found that this was not to be the case. I couldn't accept the chronic treatment anyhow. I wanted to get on with my life, take the medication, lose the weight and then think about the horrible nightmare at a later point in my life. I ballooned from a 30 to a 36 waist and suspenders. My body image was suffering and I did not know what to do with how I looked. I could no longer run. Walking up stairs caused tremendous bone-draining energy drain and fatigue.

A phenomenon occurred, before I was diagnosed, I had a biopsy. I was feeling <u>very</u> <u>well</u> but the doctor said that you are <u>doing very badly</u>; we need to put you on a regime. Now, I was feeling cruddy <u>and crummy</u> as you can get and the doctor noted that my body was <u>doing very well</u>. Go figure! And find mine while you're out there. For me this was a big dilemma, especially when I looked at myself and compared myself to what I looked like a month ago. I now know how vain that thought was and is but it is what I honestly was thinking. I was more concerned about my looks and the obesity than with this disease that was ravaging my body. I was reluctantly taking treatment and not wanting to accepting the results. The doctors were positive that they would be able to help me with this condition and resolve it. Resolve it into remission. After six months, I was weaned off the medication, I began to lose weight, my memory returned but I still had residuals in my system. I was now 185 lbs (up from 130 lbs) and my knees were literally buckling under all of the pressure. I resolved to start an exercise program to get the weight off. Walks, jogging and I started to become aware of my nutritional needs. If I was going to eat then I needed the most healthful food to me. All through out this time, I was still having Uveitis symptoms. I began to delve and research the complications Sarcoidosis presents in the eyes and how it is related to these complications. I discovered that 5% of Sarcoidosis patients that have eye involvement usually have a chronic condition. There is was right there in black and white. I found this out when my diagnosis was actually positive. I had no lung involvement, no irregular heartbeat, except for the eyes. I became more aware and alarmed that I might have the chronic form of Sarcoidosis. What should I do? Once again the tiger was staring me in the face and I had no clue as to how to contain him. The doctors cleared me…gave me a clean bill of health but I knew that I could not have recovered because I still had inflammation in my eyes. From 1987 until 1992, I had no more complications, physically, except memory loss. I just compensated for this by developing different memory loss techniques, the residual weight and Uveitis. I still was fatigued but I decided to ramp up my exercise. I still was aggressively researching everything about this disease. I became more and more leery and uneasy. I learned that every system could be affected and no one could do anything about it and there was no known cure; yet it is not contagious. At the end of the course load, I wrote a paper on Sarcoidosis. While waiting to turn our papers in one of my classmates looked at my paper, with quite some interest. I learned later on that her mother was diagnosed with Sarcoidosis and my research paper helped her to understand a little bit more of what was going on. She mentioned that her mother had Sarcoidosis a long time and they never knew what it was. It seemed to be a disease that looked like other things. They thought it was "Wandering Uterus Syndrome" or "Female Abnormalities" or "chronic Fatigue" or Lyme Disease" Earlier in the year, the mother was diagnosed, the paper helped to understand what she could do and she was able to share the devastating affects and what to expect with her mother. At this particular time, you needed to research independently and it was not openly available to everyone and it was not all in one central location. I was also elated to find out by researching my paper had some information that the National Sarcoidosis Foundation also was trying to inform people about this disease. I was a student and this paper was just temporary, like the class and life with the Sarcoidosis and so I held on to that belief.

In my research, I noted that Sarcoidosis could be equally as devastating as diabetes; it required a lot of rehabilitation. This peaked my interest in physical rehabilitation. I wondered if there were people who diagnoses were incorrect because this disease mimics others. It was more devastating in their lives now. Rehabilitation was an area that I was interested in and I pursued it after I graduated from Nursing School.

4

What Exactly Is Sarcoidosis?

The disease and the conditions that it brought on. I came to the conclusion that this was something that had future, long-term implications. It is my opinion that not many people would really know about or appreciate its potential to do harm. I didn't appreciate this fact and I had it. Interesting things would occur after I accepted having this disease; I met other people, with different degrees of Sarcoidosis. I became more aware of people who had Chronic Fatigue Syndrome, noting that the symptoms are quite like mine. Joint diseases, eye diseases and other conditions that affected the body and how different drugs interact with different systems at different times for different purposes. One of the greatest conclusions that I had to come faced to face with was that this was not some type of disease that I could ignore and treat sparingly. I had to watch it, monitor it and keep constant vigil. No more denial I came into acceptance. I had health-care professionals who recognized the disease. I was lucky. As those living with the disease know, there is no definitive etiology. And the pathology is not clear, the lineage is not clear. No one knows where it came from where it goes. Definitive though is that it is an autoimmune disease. Perplexing…if there is an inflammation in your body then there is a reaction to something. You have to figure out what there was a reaction to. But understand mainly people who were exposed to various things in the South-eastern states (I spent al lot of my child-hood in Southeaster Georgia), African-Americans, Jewish, Greek Isle, Scandinavians and some military personnel in the Gulf War (I) are all groups that have clusters of individuals with this disease. But there is no pinpoint specific as to where this disease comes from. Research for paper, doctors told me this information. Another interesting fact is that although not contagious, doctors have observed that if one person in a family has it, there is a greater chance of another person (within that same extended family) of contracting the disease. I had to be aware of the treatment modes causing other problems. Doctors didn't know how to treat it and all that was in your favor was luck because you'd either go into remission or left with a chronic situation. Bottom line is to be your best advocate and keep yourself informed of the latest studies of the disease.

Definition of Sarcoidosis

Remember the physical for the military? They diagnosed me with an irregularity on the x-ray and enlarged lymph nodes. That is the first telltale sign. The doctor did not know what it was…so it isn't true that the military will just take any living, breathing soul. You actually have to be physically fit. That was good to know although it was not comforting at the time. The other symptom in 1984 was the pinkeye every severe case. I only had a previous less severe case of pinkeye. I am extremely ultra hygienic and very clean, orderly person but I thought that maybe I had gotten it from someone. What was fascinating about this case of Pink-eye" was that it transferred to the other eye the next week. At this time my eyes were extremely light sensitive; even the picture that I to take for my job, the flashbulb hurt. I thought this was extremely abnormal. I had never heard of that. I self treated this one. It went away. I then started to note that I had scaly legs. I had no clue as to what was going on and I thought that they were the "ashy" variety and would be cured with extra thick, moisturizing lotion. I thought it was dry skin. I did notice that more and more skin would peel off and no other person in my life had encountered this kind of peeling.

Remember the visit to the optometrist? What he saw and described to me was amazing. He saw a star-like configuration in my pupils. And it was supposed to be a round configuration. Remember the ophthalmologist, his diagnosis was Uveitis (a basic inflammation of the eye-ball). He tried to explain to me the condition further and offered to see me over time for a reduced fee. I didn't understand what information was being related to me. He was actually letting me know that my eyes would get worse and that I would probably need to see him for the rest of my life. And I thought that he was offering me a reduced fee because he liked me! It was charming! This doctor was the first one to use the term Sarcoidosis. He defined it for me. It was an autoimmune disease and something like Lupus. He didn't go into how bad it would be for me eventually. I should have been thankful that it was diagnosed then. I felt like a healthy person.

I had to admit there was then a problem with my endurance. I pegged this as being a part of growing old and being inactive but in my late twenties? However, I found that my shortness of breath was to be much more troublesome than I thought. I started to do more research and found that there was a possibility of lung involvement. At the time, I was smoking and I attributed the shortness of breath to this filthy habit. I was still quite athletic at this time. During this time period, I had no other new symptoms.

In New York (1987) during my Nursing School years. I underwent a physical examination and it was a healthy review. I anticipated having all of the previous symptoms and there was nothing that was exposed so I started a new exercise program. For the most part, everything as normal until the Nursing School clinical. This was when the Instructor confirmed that my pulse was irregular and strongly encouraged me get an affidavit saying that it was not life threatening. This was also about the time when basketball player Len Bias died allegedly from complications regarding his heartbeat so everyone was becoming extra-sensitive and aware of this condition. The Instructors did not want a health-crisis on their hands to say the least. My ophthalmologist also thought more aggressive treatment for my eyes, was needed. I was completely swamped with studying. Case in point, I had trouble noticing a voluptuous woman, walking towards me. This fact, in my mind, supported the doctor's view. We had to get serious about the eyes.

I started my medical regime with the cortical steroid, Prednisone. Most people with Sarcoidosis are very familiar with this medication whether it is Solumetrol® or Preforte® but it is very familiar in its weight-inducing capabilities. I went from a healthy weight to unhealthy weight gain. I felt the fat in the back of my neck. I didn't feel that I was progressing but the doctors said that I was. Prednisone, in my opinion, only worked to do and to alleviate some symptoms of the disease and the proportion of other things that exist with Sarcoidosis, to me, outweighs whatever benefit that Prednisone provides but people seem to think that something is better than nothing. The side effects were horrible to me...a raw deal.

My experience has been gratefully different from others. Other people go from doctor to doctor trying to get the disease diagnosed. I was my biggest obstacle. It is a multi-system disease but it manifests itself as a single symptom in the beginning. My single symptom, as you recall, was the ashy skin and the problem with my vision. As I would lose the ability to exercise, I would get fatigued; other people were thinking that it was Lyme disease. In New York, this was definitely a possibility. Because of my Lung involvement, some family members mistakenly thought that it was the contagious Tuberculosis. Some of them also began to spread the rumor that I had HIV-AIDs. I was trying to disseminate information about my condition as quickly as possible to dissipate any type of fear that my loved ones might have and yet, I still endured the questioning glances and "unknowing" stares and false whispers and rumors but what was even more ignorant, the mistreatment and plain mass hysteria, all within my own family! Doctors do not diagnose conditions as related to this disease as in Asthma induced by Sarcoidosis, or COPD as induced by Sarcoidosis they diagnose it almost in a vacuum. Indeed some of the above mentioned conditions do occur on their own but when Sarcoidosis is a remote possibility, then further investigation is indeed warranted. I had to enlighten the health-care professionals as well as others around me about the exact cause of these other things.

5

Managing the Condition/ Disease—What I do

I couldn't make that real transition from a cold area and I have a wicked cough. By the time I went through this whole litany of things I had, people still questioned whether I was telling the truth. This had to be a lie and that I was covering up for some other horrid disease as if this wasn't bad enough to have. It's possible that he has something else. When I would gain weight, it would hurt. People would say, in their ignorance of Prednisone effects, "Boy are you eating like a pig." Here I am starving myself so I could reduce the weight and still going through the inquisition posed by loved ones. Here I am getting weaker and their advice to me was to cut down on eating the cheesecakes. "If you didn't drink that chocolate milk then you wouldn't be getting so fat." When I explained that I would get larger because of the medication, going through the litany again I would get the glazed over looks and the same retort would come out of their mouths about my fork and knife problem. "You just need will power. That's your only problem." Things like, staying out of the sun…Do you have a skin problem? They would go to the wild extreme in thought, nearing the irrational. They would take a little bit of knowledge and make some very unwise assumptions about my condition and me. Folks start looking at you like you are strange and to be honest, you start looking at yourself and questioning whether you are indeed strange yourself.

Gradually, I had to rely on the expertise of the researcher and put aside my doubts and say "yes" this is Sarcoidosis and that I have it and probably will have to educate people who come into contact with me. You cannot think it away or use positive thoughts. Prayer works though. Positive reasoning was not going to cause this thing to go away. It had to be acted upon. Attack it headfirst and do not shun from the responsibility. And of course, the greatest enemy was myself. I had to quit denying that I was the same person that I was before diagnosis. Something else was different. Whatever history I had, athletic, football, wrestling, laying out in sun and field work all things of the past—-memories. Right now a new reality, and new existence. My denial had cost possible delay in treatment. I had lung involvement and that was diagnosed eye involvement, weight gain—-an issue of image and vanity for me. But there was so much pressure in my knees and joints causing me to be in constant pain. There is always a dull pain anyway. My knees are always hurting anyway and if I run or move the wrong way or put too much trauma on my knees they will swell. This issue was something that I could grab hold of mentally and I could fix it.

6

Drug Interactions

A fortunate case in where we live in a society where many types of conditions can be handled or cured by the use of drugs. However, we must be vigilant and know that drugs can do something helpful or can be harmful. At this time, there is only one real medical regime for the treatment of Sarcoidosis and that is Corticosteroids and one in particular Prednisone. These have somewhat devastation long-term effects. The thing that has changed since my diagnosis is the definition of Sarcoidosis. They now say that it is a long-term or chronic condition. It is no longer considered Acute. This is very different and the consequences are serious. In 87 after the biopsy, I began taking 60 milligrams of Prednisone. He described the side affects, slightly weight, and gain, no sun exposure, possible liver and kidney complications but not to worry because I would only be using it for the short term. (Six months). The main reason to be on it is the lung involvement; once I went into the hospital the lungs were involved. It is really to the benefit of patients and advocates and individuals to always question their doctors and do research themselves. We can have the best doctors, but sometimes they are over confident and flippant and take for granted a lot of stuff that we do not take for granted in the lay world. The doctor just mentioned the "Slight" weight gain and short-term complications but he did not explain the full consequences. It was not explained as to how to take three different types of medications. Take them all at once or half during the day or evening. I immediately took all 60 grams at once. Those with Sarcoidosis can imagine what fun this was. All of sudden "slight weight" gain was like a "little bit pregnant'. I did not understand the voracious appetite that I did acquire and my hips and joints were very sensitive. I had to be very careful when moving because if my foot got caught on the carpet, there was a possibility that I would pull my hip out of place. And if I pulled my hip out of place, yikes—-excruciating pain. The joints were more fragile. I also noticed the memory loss. Remember I was going to school and studying and I could not understand why I couldn't recall the facts for exams and such. The drug does two good things and 20 bad things. Sarcoidosis patients are very limited in what they can do; the parameters are clearly defined for me. I tried experimenting with vitamin c, melatonin neither worked for me. You really have to research and advocate for yourself. Some doctors' philosophy is that this is what you will have to go through, get over it, see you next week. You have to prepare yourself for the regime of living with this stuff. I am a free thinker and open to new medical experiments. My memory loss, I compensated by doing phonics and making copious lists.

I am a Southern Baptist and we teach in church that some people can hear spirits talking. I was very open to hearing the voice of God; however the voices I began hearing were NOT god-like! They were very irritating. The television started talking to me and it wasn't on. This was a point of extreme concern to me. It was trying to tell me to do some unchristian-like things (definitely psychosis), non-productive. Everyone has a problem with traffic and I was stuck in traffic and I had this irresistible urge to ram the car in from of me. Fortunately, I was able to tell myself that this was not rational. Upon walking on the street, things would come into my mind and I would wonder how they got there. I also noticed that I was actually hearing words. I did some more research and found that Prednisone does cause psychosis but they do not describe what you will go through. It would have been helpful to know before I befriended the Purple People. Insomnia is a huge side affect. Sometimes your body will force you to take a rest whether you like it or not. That caused me some minor concern, although since I was studying, I didn't think that was too big a negative. I could take a sleeping pill and that helped me to go to sleep but the sleep was not restful. After all this time, we still only have that one option for this condition. The drug also causes irritability. When you're trying to think rationally. The simple fact of life of waiting in a doctor's office caused me great anxiousness. I could not take it. I was having violent thoughts and tendencies. The doctor prescribed a different way of taking the drug. I took half of the Prednisone in the morning and half in the evening. We would live with it like that. That helped a little but it also increased the weight gain, the thorn in my vanity's side. I was outgrowing my clothes overnight. During this period, the voices were nicer and conversations were there but I recognized that they were not real. The regime was reduced to wean me off the medication. For this initial period, there were no problems or complications. In latter years, of course more problems surfaced.

I am no longer being weaned off of the drug instead I have switched to a maintenance program. Maintenance…just like cars. The pulmonologist weaned me off the medication after the initial six months. He said that he saw significant increase in my lung capacity. I was still sensitive to the sun and I still had a voracious appetite. From 1987 to 1990. I was placed on a maintenance dose for my eyes. There was always a complication with my eyes. The disease never went into total remission because it would always manifest itself into my eyes. Over the years, that has been a continual focal point. It seemed that I had taken a magic bullet. It was still dormant in my eyes. Over the years, I have had the occasion to travel to different towns, in 96 I went to Dallas, Texas and I experienced severe breathing problems. The barometric pressure was extremely high. I had a real serious outbreak in the area because I could not breathe. I had to be hospitalized and was placed on the regime again. In the hospital, they give you Solumetrol®, when you're out, that drug is not available. You have to push for this stuff and Prednisone is more readily available. You have to eat to prevent ulceration with this medication. The disease causes calcium waste and therefore I had to take calcium supplements. Research now indicates that Sarcoidosis patients have an extremely high level of calcium in their blood stream. I do not know if I was doing myself any favors. What do you think?

7

Pros and Cons

The initial critical points about the pros and cons would be the expectations. In 1987 to 1996, for me was this was an acute situation, it was viewed with more enthusiasm, Prednisone was the silver bullet and would take away all my problems and I could be rid of this monster. That wasn't the case. In 1996, it would be 10 years that I was dealing with this situation. I had a chronic condition. The only drugs available were the steroids. High doses of melatonin was not useful, high doses of vitamin c was not useful, there were no other drugs. One thing that had to be combined with the drug regime was how to modify the drug. As mentioned before, a complication from medication was insomnia, so one had to take some type of sleeping pill. Well, I found out that I had to take something stronger, like a tranquilizer. Ambien® works however it only lasts two hours in my case. So you had to modify how you take it. I had to take anti-depressants, whichever one should I take? Zoloft © or Effexer ©. Effexer© is a titrated drug, therefore you can't come off of Prednisone quickly. You 're sustained by drugs and they are all interacting with each other and you've got a roller coaster of chemicals going off in your body. And if anybody, any drugs bumps into each other, you are in a world of trouble. The same with the other complications because of the long term use, sometimes you are forced to take insulin. That in and of itself complicates matters, you'll have to determine what units to take and what time of day and where you're going to take it, where to inject yourself either in the stomach or the shoulder. When you come off to go on something like Glucophage®, how many calories do you take in? Right now I am on an 1800-calorie restriction. I know others that are on a 1500-calorie restriction. You have to interact with your sugars. With African Americans, you have to be careful of being iron saturated at the same time, iron spillage and calcium spillage, which leads to potassium loss, which could cause an irregular heartbeat and fatigue. It becomes a real tightrope to walk not knowing what you can and cannot do with Sarcoidosis. With my eye involvement at one time I had to use Diomox ®

because the pressure in my eyes exacerbated the condition and caused an acidotic condition in my body, I couldn't breathe, so no matter how much iron I got, it was useless for conversion of oxygen. The body has to be pH balanced. So now you have to determine if you can handle this with a food supplement or pill. My particular problem was that at this time, the doctors did not know about an alkaline imbalance. The only things that they knew, concerning the pills, were that they had something containing charcoal that I could swallow that would stop the acid in my stomach but that was a palliative product. It wasn't doing anything for the body condition. Once again, we have to be our best advocate finding out regimes and what works. Because of the skin problems, I used vitamins A, B and E and usually I use Ester-C about 2,000 mg for collagen building. I thought that it was helpful but at time progresses it becomes a little bit cumbersome keeping everything in proper perspective.

If you have a companion, spouse or other loved one helping you, you need to give them extra consideration and kindness and care because this chaotic complicated schedule becomes a part of their lives also. I know when I forget something; the weight is all on my wife to remember what to do. It is imperative that you can trust or learn to trust that person. It is also imperative that they take on the responsibility knowing all of the ramifications. Because my memory is impaired when it comes to certain things, like my eye medicine, times I took it. I recall a story that I was telling my sister. I was speaking with her and I had placed the code to retrieve my messages from the phone in a certain place so that I would remember it when I forgot where I placed it. I forgot the number and the place so I had to wait around six hours for the Prednisone effects to diminish so I could remember my telephone number and how to access the messages. This underscores the importance of active awareness of what the drugs are doing to us.

Another thing that I did not want to be caught up in was that spiral drug interactions. I knew this was the case with the heart condition. With the case of the Sarcoidosis, it causes the tissue to conduct the electrical pulses and therefore the EKG readings were off the scale. I was placed on the monitor and went home. The hospital personnel were calling me every hour trying to admit me to the hospital because they were sure that I was having a heart attack. I had to convince them that I was doing fine, there were no problems. When I did get there, they examined me several times, because it looked like I should be having a heart attack but that wasn't the case. I had to keep myself from being caught up in the loop. They wanted to give me medications for congestion, and then another med for something else and then you're caught up in the spiral. Right now they're giving me a medication for high blood pressure. They say it's for high blood pressure but my doctor says they want to always check my kidneys. Drugs that are given for blood pressure usually are diuretics caused the fluids to leave your body and don't cause a congestive situation. It's not going to do anything for the blood pressure, my reading is 110 over 80 but she wants me to have kidney functions that are not hampered and that's the major reason for that medication but if I continue to take these drugs I am going to have some problems. Why should I take it when I don't have high blood pressure and the doctor tells me to take it as a precautionary measure? I could understand, but if I take it, the diuretics will drain all of my electrolytes and I will be fatigued. Remember that I still have a condition of calcium waste. This causes a possibility of an irregular heartbeat and muscle fatigue. Drugs, they are beneficial but you have to take them knowing what you are doing to your body and be your best advocate.

Everything is being filtered through the liver and all the toxic chemicals going through you. In the hospital, you get antibiotics that are killing bacteria; one needs a pro-biotic to reintroduce the good flora that's being killed. That reintroduction of good flora helps with your digestion, counter-acts the acid tic or alkaline situation with your digestion. Everything is interacting with every thing and everything is being filtered through the kidneys and liver. The liver and kidneys are very important and they are involved in Sarcoidosis. They are getting worn out with the chemicals. Sometimes they just fade out.

Right now I have Diabetes caused by Sarcoidosis, so I have some kidney, cholesterol, anti-depressants, Prednisone and Eye pressure medication. It's like I'm eating a handful or Raisinets © when I take my medication. All of these pills to treat every possible scenario and issues in my body that have all been caused by Prednisone. I can't put my finger on it but something is not quite right about this. I just was informed that I could develop kidney stones, which is more painful kidney stones or not having kidney function? And those are some of the choices that we all have to make with our medical regime. Take the drugs and blow out your organs or the alternative. It would be different if there were more medical regimes available to us but unfortunately we have only those two and we have to determine how we can exist within them.

There is a big issue with the lung involvement with the use of oxygen. My case, I am doing really well as long as I am sitting in one position but as soon as I move, I have a problem with oxygen. I was living with my sister, in Dallas, and it was a struggle every night to get up and go to the bathroom. It would take me ten minutes before I could use the restroom because I would run out of oxygen. I even set up my bed in the bathroom at one point. Because of the effort that it took to get from the floor to the toilette was so exhausting. I sat down on the couch thinking that if I sat down, then I'd have a better chance at breathing. Slowly creeping up and trying to make me pay the toll for what I had done, in my lungs, attacking it. I sat up thinking that I'd have the best space for my diaphragm on the floor. Could not breathe, my heart started to beat faster and faster, I' couldn't breathe and all that I had done was to walk from one room to the next! I grabbed the side of the couch. I cried Lord, Lord why are you torturing me like this, why are you doing this to me, why don't you just kill me, Lord because I could not breathe and I fell to the floor. I could feel the urine leaking from me. I knew that was the sign for death, the last thing that happens in the body is the loss of bodily functions before you die. It was so desperate and I surrendered and knew that I would die and then…. the air miraculously began to filter into my lungs. Oh sweet breath. I was faced down on the floor, but I could breathe. My heart was racing and bursting out of my chest, but I could breathe. All of this because I wanted to walk from one room to the other. I thought to myself, I've GOT to get to the hospital and off the floor but how could I. The floor became my home. This is my daily struggle.

Over the years, I started seeing the breakdown in my system. Specifically, I noted. problems with the acute situation in the year 2000. Then I started to notice more breathing complications, I could deal with that, but the scarring of my lungs. The onset of diabetes snuck up on me. All of a sudden, I seemed to be very thirsty and it struck me that I was urinating a lot and had no energy so I did think of it as a possibility. I went to the hospital and was diagnosed with Diabetes; my sugar level was at 800 units. It was reported to me that this was related to the Sarcoidosis. Strange things happen…when I tried to reduce the amount of Prednisone from 40 grams to 20 g, the degree of Diabetes was reduced. I've been maintaining a Sugar level of 110–120 consistently as I've reduced the amount of Prednisone that I'm using. It's directly related to how your body functions.

I found that the use of has an interesting effect when you are dependent on Oxygen and sometimes the lungs need to be exercised independently of the Oxygen, induced flow. It is not helpful to your body to be so depended on medication but the double-edge sword is just feeling better with the medical regime than without. I have to employ a multi-vitamin. You have to find a good one and something with a supplement for Joint support. I need Calcium and iron supplement? At times I have used Gatorade® and apple juice or apple cider and it caused my sugar level to go sky high. In my quest to eat healthy another thing that I found strange, I found that the hallucinations will come on with high dosages of Tylenol and Ibuprofen and I found that they seemed to cause hallucinations in conjunction with my other medications. My wife was worried. My sister asked me to better monitor yourself, "because if you open up your bathroom and you have tiny men talking to you, it could lead to problems and especially if t you are talking to them". Pretty soon they were laughing at me but soon they would turn on me. They were not green they were purple.

I had to find out for myself what was working and what wasn't. The other part of my medical regime is to monitor the oxygen intake that I have. I did not know that oxygen is designated as a drug and you have to have a prescription for it. And you have to qualify for it. What! Can't you see I'm almost dead—-it still isn't good enough? When I didn't have to take all these medicines–I am depending on that happening again. This is supposed to be a teaching college and the dearth of information was not there. The respiratory therapists, that I've encountered, have a particular irritating attitude to me. You are on oxygen and they will test your oxygen saturation rate, of course it is good when you are attached! Do they not think that they should test when you are not hooked up! This is not an efficient way to measure. The very effort of just sitting on the side of the bed was overwhelming. It would cause me to go into the hyperventilation. It was so horrible and I had to work with the nurses that would know to give me something to relax my muscles so that I would continue with whatever machinations they were subjecting me to. Just moving one foot was so painful; many times I thought I'd rather pee in the bed than to risk getting up. But I knew that I'd have to get up to change the bed linens and that would be even more painful than just holding it through the pain. That thought kept me going! Another thing, be aware of what their doing to you. You don't want them to give you a D5W in the hospital.

I find the strange thing that has happened, the medicines have become a part of my life. I attempted to fast and found that I could not do that. I have a schedule well I think that medications are better absorbed at 7:00 am. If I wait until 9:00 am I will be in pain, I have to take the Prednisone. I can not skip a day. Some people can get on and off of it. I can not do that, I have to have my 20 mg, my joints hurt, breathing is interfered with. I am trapped with my anti-depressants. I am being turned into a slave for the medicine. Which they say is to combat the condition. I just can't figure out which is more devastating, the regime or the disease. Some natural medicines are too pricey for me on my fixed budget. I believe in the Grapeseed Extract. I was taking Gingko but I've stopped.

I must get out of the house. It is part of my medical regime. I must get out of the house and be as active as much as I can. Washing the dishes is therapeutic for me and adds to me feelings of being worthwhile. All of the agencies have branded me as being not worthwhile, NOT VIABLE. I must also keep busy, keep active and knowledgeable and try to have the best day that I can. I drink filtered water and do not mess with sodas. I have modified the Atkins® diet for me. I must eat at a certain time; I must actually write it down because Prednisone makes you forget. I eat Vegetables, green leafy for the calcium. Part of the disease is that you waste calcium so you need to replenish them besides, my wife cooks some delicious greens, turkey and chicken. I have to remember that I can not forget my eating plan. I can not lapse and get over a certain weight, it is not good for my knees, the extra weight. I have to exercise as much as I can, and staying positive, no matter what. I can not get depressed over something that I am going to be successful at. My higher power has deemed this to be so.

8

Eating Plan

We have heard from the "experts" that eating the correct foods can aide in maintaining a healthy body. It is indeed true especially for those of us with food sensitivities brought on or exacerbated by Sarcoidosis. The following pages contain helpful recipes that aid me in my quest to maintain this body for as long as the time that I'm given. Please feel free to change them in any way according to your tastes and dietary needs. For nutrition the blender is a good friend. You can place cooked, steamed or raw vegetables, fruit etc. inside and combine to create the correct vitamin laced meal. Some are better tan others at this task, it's up to you to find one that will be your helper in the kitchen.

Pantry Essentials

Tofu (medium) Follow my special recipe for preparation or you'll never attempt to eat this fantastic food again. Think yummy, with recipe. Think wallpaper paste WITHOUT the recipe.

Garlic (helpful to the immune system)
Water
Apples (vitamin c, control diabetes, has fiber)
Celery (known to reduce high blood pressure, great source or potassium)
Onions (reduces inflammation, relieves congestion, helps to lower blood pressure)
Cucumbers
Watermelon (helps to keep blood pressure low)
Chicken
Beans (butter, navy, lima, green)
Mustard Greens (protection against vision loss)
Rutabaga

Kale ((helps control blood pressure, protect against vision loss)
Tilapia (fish) (reduces lung inflammation, magnesium rich)
Salmon (contains helpful vitamin e)
Broccoli (boosts immunity, has beta carotene, vitamin c and calcium)
Eggplant
Cabbage (lowers risk of cataracts, helps to prevent some cancers and heart disease)
Sweet potatoes (helps to preserve memory, control diabetes)
Eggs (protein)
Pecans (protects against heart disease)
Field peas ((relieve cold symptoms)
Blackberries or blueberries (protection against cataracts and reduces infection)
Peaches, nectarines (good fiber and vitamin c)
Oatmeal (fiber)
Grits (staple of the south)
Popcorn (not with a lot of butter or salt)
Cilantro
Rosemary
Zucchini
Olive Oil (can help to lower cholesterol, protects heart)
Corn (can boost energy levels)
Pears
Flaxseed (1/4 cup sprinkled on cereal)
Supplemental vitamins (A, E and D)
Filtered water (can be gotten free, from your sink)
Ionizer (air)

This is just a suggested list. Some of these foods may change depending if you have Diabetes as a result of the medication that you're taking. This is the case with me. I have referenced the nutritive values from several sources. When in doubt, please speak with your doctor.

Everything fresh must be washed to include "organically" grown, to get rid of spores and any other airborne items traveling on it. You can spice things up with a little bit of vinegar or other powdered spices that have no additional salt (or MSG) in them. I know some of you are curious as to why I placed the ionizer at the bottom of the food list. It is placed here so you'll know that it too is essential to filtering out airborne particles in the environment around your home. It is very helpful. Also remember that studies show that patients with Sarcoidosis have high amounts of calcium in their bloodstreams so be mindful of foods that will cause you to leech more calcium or give you too much.

Recipes

Enjoyable Tofu

12 oz firm tofu (cut into small cubes)
1/3 cup teriyaki sauce
1 ½ tbs. butter
2 tbs garlic powder

Combine all ingredients (except garlic powder) in a skillet. Fry for 5 minutes. The tofu should be firm and slightly beige or golden brown on some sides. Sprinkle garlic powder on and stir for 30 more seconds. Remove from heat, drain and serve. (This recipe can be used to add tofu to any other dish that you desire.)

Parmesan Eggplant with Tofu

You will need: 1 eggplant, sliced into ½ width (about 8)
½ teas. Salt
1 large onion, sliced
1 head of garlic, crushed
Prepare tofu (use recipe above, only cut in thin flat slices).

Lightly spray a baking pan with non-stick oil. Place all ingredients in pan making sure to layer eggplant and tofu on top of each other. Bake at 400 degrees for 40 minutes. Take out of over and sprinkle top with parmesan cheese. Let stand for 2 minutes and then serve.

Kale, Collard and Mustard Green Mix

Use fresh green combination or can use the canned greens (drain the liquid to reduce the salt)
2 tbs of olive oil
1 small onion
vinegar to taste

Sauté onion in olive oil until slightly brown. Remove from stove. Place green mixture in large pot, with 1 cup of water bring to a boil over medium heat. Add onion/olive oil mixture. Stir, turn down heat and let simmer for 15 more minutes. Add vinegar and serve warm.

Broccoli Scones

Fresh broccoli (can use bag of frozen chopped broccoli)
4 eggs
1 cup bread crumbs
¼ tsp. salt and pepper
½ pad of butter

Steam broccoli in butter. (2 minutes, don't overcook). Let cool and remove from heat. Place in blender and puree 30 seconds. Combine eggs, bread crumbs, salt and pepper with the broccoli puree in a bowl. Roll into patties and fry until a thin crust has formed on both sides. Serve warm

Healthy, Any Time Salsa

2 cucumbers, cut and drained
1 cup plain yogurt
1/2 teas. Kosher salt
1 small onion
3 tbs. freshly chopped cilantro
1 tbs. lime juice
pinch of pepper
(optional, 2 small cherry tomatoes, chopped and drained)

Combine all ingredients. Chill in refrigerator for 30 minutes. Serve on any meats and especially fish.

Burritos

3 chicken breast, grilled or baked sliced thin strips
5 tbs cilantro
1 large Vidalia ® onion or a yellow one, diced
2 tbs. lime juice
2 garlic cloves (minced)
5 tortillas
Pepper (1 green and 1 red, sliced)
Lettuce (try other varieties not just iceberg)

Warm tortillas in oven (250 degrees for 15 minutes) or microwave (10 seconds on high). Place onions and peppers in a skillet and sauté until onions are brown. Add garlic cloves and lime juice for 1 minute. Remove from stove and set aside. Combine cilantro and lettuce. Place all ingredients onto the warm tortillas, roll and eat.

Eggplant Spread

½ cup olive oil
1 tsp minced garlic
1 tsp minced basil leaves
¼ cup lemon juice
2 small eggplants (sliced into 5 or 6 thin portions)

Combine all ingredients and place in bag. Marinate for 4 hours. Take out and place on non-stick pan. Broil 3 minutes on each side. Place in blender and chop then puree for 15 seconds or until the mixture appears smooth. Spoon into a small bowl or onto a small plate. Eat with toasted whole wheat bread or crackers. It is also great with celery.

Scrumptious Salmon

4 six oz. salmon fillet (skin off)
¼ teas. Salt
pepper
1 tbs. olive oil
Heinz® 57 sauce
Basil for each fillet
1 teas. Teriyaki® sauce (rub on each side of salmon before cooking)

Salt salmon. Let sit for 30 minutes. Season with pepper, basil. Heat olive oil (medium heat, non-stick skillet). Fry salmon (may also be grilled or broiled) for 5 minutes on each side. Serve hot.

Creamy Broccoli Soup

Broccoli stems (frozen)
½ cup of prepared broccoli soup
1/3 cup cream
1 tbs. olive oil
¼ cup of warm water.

Steam broccoli until soft. Place all ingredients in the pot with the broccoli. Bring to a boil. Remove from heat. Place everything in your blender and whip for 20 seconds. Pour into bowls and serve warm.

Reflections

I remember times of being lost when I did not have a reference point. Standing still and listening trying to feel, to pick up the slightest indication of how to proceed. I remember studying animals that were rejected by the pack. They would walk towards the pack very humbling so, so submissive, so wanting to be obviously needed by the other members. And the other pack members would let them in but there were times of rejection for whatever reason, that particular animal was left out, left to wander around. Go to another place and be run off again. It seemed to have some kind of mark, some kind of indicator which made it undesirable to the others. In many ways for me, Sarcoidsosis has made me a marked person. And sometimes as a marked person it has both the effect of making me desirable and undesirable at the same time. But I am very pleased that I was raised with a view that I have a fundamental idea of who I am and I really don't need the pack or at least lot of stuff. But as the song goes, "everybody needs somebody sometimes to love" and when you get to the point where you do not need someone to love at least from my point that's when you become lost. When I am on my own thinking to myself, talking with myself about things that should be a two person conversation. Many times Sarcoidosis has caused me to mark myself and not want to be part of any one's group. Because I get tired of the process. I get tired of it mentally, of being aware of who I'm with. Are they sick? Do they have a hidden diseases, shaking people's hands, what hygiene do they have? It is fickle and picky but it is necessary for me.

In my mind, you get an invitation to a party, do I want to go. What is there waiting for me? How do I take it? When I rode the bus, I know longer do, this guy wanted to talk with me. He had a cold and was sneezing and in my mind I saw the big germ molecules spewing out of him. I would move and he would follow me to sit by me. He just wanted to talk but trying to fend off people and other disease makes me unable to be able to afford to talk with you. You might give me a cold and it would lead to so many complications for me. This is totally out of my character, I love talking to anyone, family or complete strangers. I did not want to take the risk of endangering my life by just talking to you. That sounds cruel. Before I had this degree of Sarcoidosis, I was able to deal with people with varying conditions. Patients need to be touched. They need to have human contact. For me, having to protect myself at this level has caused me to alienate and cut off a very important need for human contact.

I remember asking myself how does someone become a recluse. Now I know, I had the makings of a Howard Hughes with out the money, maids and mansion. I am becoming that person. For whatever reason, for caution, fear…you close yourself away from human interaction for what you consider is a higher need….self preservation. At what cost?

I was given a choice to have a heart, lung replacement. I knew of the requirements but my decision had been made. A brand new set, but you're placing those new organs into a body that is riddled with the Sarcoidosis. Ultimately they would be affected and infected. I passed on this. Someone else could use them. More pressing for me to regain my sight. I miss this sensory the most. I miss viewing the new car lines out. I wasn't interested in any other organs. I could take control of this one decision. This disease has been with me for forty years and slowly ravaged me. I used to watch the boxing greats, I liked the strategy where some boxers slowly destroy the other by affecting him slowly and overall until you're able to knock them out. I likened it to Sarcoidosis. It has taken on a life of it's own and is my opponent. It doesn't care who it attacks. It has an affinity for Scandinavians, for Japanese people, for southern blacks. It can reshape itself for different ways. For some it affects different parts, acute or long term chronic. For me it has claimed my life and I have been living each six months by God's grace. This is the time period that each new doctor gives me after their initial assessment. I understand that the fight is already (just like a Tyson boxing fight) over for me but I still have no time to die.

I am in the category, the 5% that are killed by the disease outright. Albeit slow and agonizing but at least there won't be any surprises. I was fortunate to be diagnosed early and not having my disease misdiagnosed as hysterics or chronic fatigue syndrome or Lupus.

Today the diagnosis is not so invasive, the old test was whether the problems warranted minor surgery. The main problem is to me, having this Sarcoidosis has closed me up to include the blindness. I had to change my persona. For me that is a real major issue. I always thought that I knew who I was, it has caused me to change how I interact with people. With people that have hygienic challenges I find it repulsive to be around. This limits my interaction capabilities. I try to avoid large crowds because of the chances of contracting colds or other germs. Yes, I admit this is classic paranoia. But, as I mentioned before, life has indeed changed for me. There are other deadly virus which are out there and because of my nursing background, I am hyper aware of their affects.

It is very important to live near a town that can help you maintain and or enjoy the quality of life. The town that I live in is not so technically advanced. The mentality is like this (disease) is another world. I have to tell them about health aids that I need to maintain myself and these are old aids in the science world. These people do not have a clue and do not feel any urgency to get one. It feels as if it is am imposition for them to be getting the information from me because then they will have to actually DO something constructive for me. This is also the place where I was told that I am not a "viable" human being. This is the system that I and others are fighting. I am blind, have limited mobility and they do not want to provide me with the training necessary to actually live in my house, to be a little independent. Where is the support for the basics of life here? Why is this this way in the 21st century. I am having to teach myself just like millions of others. I've had many incidences of mistaking butter for ice cream. How do I brush my teeth now? Where are the classes or health professionals to teach me to live and to continue to pursue life and liberty. This is a pathetic, shameful fact of life in this town I call home; Macon, Georgia.

I want to feel that I can still take care of the little things, to make decisions for myself, to go, to feel, to experience. If you have a disease such as this, no money and limited support then you are stuck with that unless you fight and cause the changes that need to be. This is the sad fact in this town and millions of others in America. We've got to keep our voices heard. We've got to keep letting people know that you can not ignore us. You've got to be open to feel, to love and to help, to create opportunities for people that need it.

When you have a definite, finite number of years, months, days to live it seems as if that's when you realize how many more things you need to do on this earth. God gives every person a finite time to accomplish their mission and some of us get to be more aware of it ticking by. Since my diagnosis, I have wasted some precious time but it was all worth it to giggle and flirt with women, eat yummy cheesecakes, White Castle burgers, searching for 501 Bose speakers and following my favorite soap "The Young and the Restless". And yet I have wasted no time in filling my life with fruitful pursuits and interesting people. Trips to Israel to walk where my Lord and Savior walked as he expressed God's passion for us. A wonderful journey to Colorado Springs, Colorado to see America's mountain, Pikes Peak. A walk to the podium to accept my nursing degree. A walk down the aisle to meet my bride. Numerous forays to churches to set up mentor relationships and outreach programs. Entering the arduous tunnel that is the Master's degree program. Beautiful road trips to Thomasville, Georgia (the City of Roses of the South). Lovely treks up I-95 to the city that doesn't sleep and the state of my birth. Countless drives to the rehabilitation center to fight for the services that I need to live. There are many more adventures and things that I must fit into the allotted 6 months that the doctors have given me. Let's see how many more the Lord allows me to have.

I encourage you take the beautiful trips that you have always wanted to take, come high water. I encourage you to continue to participate fully in life and affect positive change for your little world. I encourage you to stand with me and speak up for those of us that are presented with a lion's share of obstacles. Let us know that we are indeed, a viable human being, a precious child of God. Take our hand and ask "How can I help you make this the best day that you can have?" Journey on with the months of grace that you have been given.

Glossary (Webster's Dictionary)

Ambien™—a drug used to help with sleeping problems.

Biopsy—the study of tissue taken from a living organism,

Diomox™—blood pressure medication, lowers eye pressure by reducing amount of water

Diuretics—a substance tending to increase discharge of urine from the body

COPD—Chronic Obstructive Pulmonary Disease

Effexer™—a drug used to combat depression.

Palliative—to make less intense or severe

Pink-eye—an acute contagious conjunctivitis, marked by inflamed eyelids and eyeballs

Sarcoid—pertaining to or resembling flesh

Sarcoidosis—an auto-immune disease of unknown origin marked by the formation of granulomatous lesions esp. in the liver, lungs, skin and lymph nodes.

Uvea—the pigmented vascular layer of the eye comprising the iris, ciliary body & choroids

Uveitis—inflammation of the uvea

Prednisone©—cortisone, used as an anti-inflammatory agent for treating arthritis

Solumetrol™—liquid Prednisome©

MSG—monosodium glutamate

Titration—determination of the concentration of a substance in solution by add-ing to it a standard agent of known concentration in carefully measured amounts until a reaction of definite and known proportion is complete, as shown by a color change of by electrical measurent, followed by calculation of the unknown concentration.

Zoloft™—drug used to help with depression.

0-595-34072-5